Social Cognitive Theory, Research, & Practice in Integrative Healthcare

Dr. Lisa Marie Portugal, PhD, EdD
The Leadership Architect

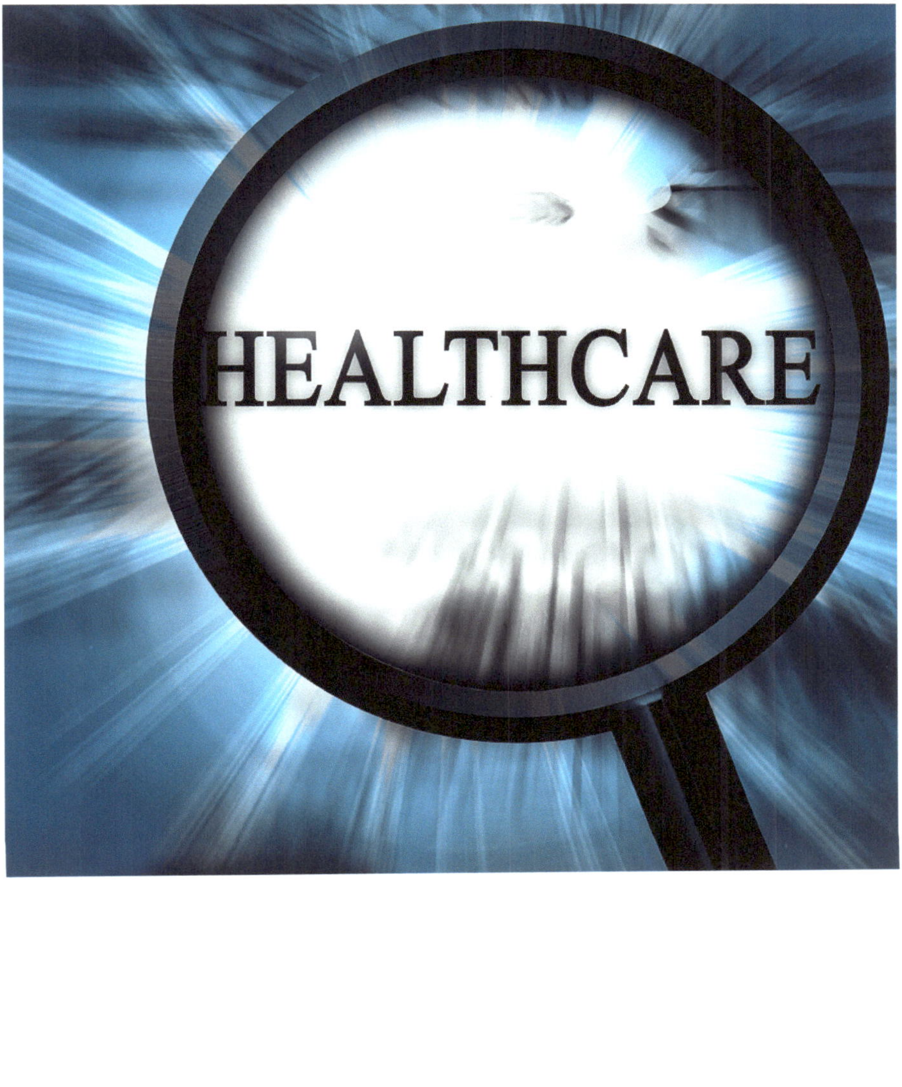

Social Cognitive Theory, Research, & Practice in Integrative Healthcare

Copyright © December 14, 2020 by Dr. Lisa Marie Portugal, PhD, EdD
All rights reserved under copyright conventions.

Published in the United States by Dr. Lisa Marie Portugal, PhD, EdD
The Leadership Architect

Library of Congress Cataloguing-in-Publication data is available
ISBN 978-1974186419
Printed in the United States
First Edition

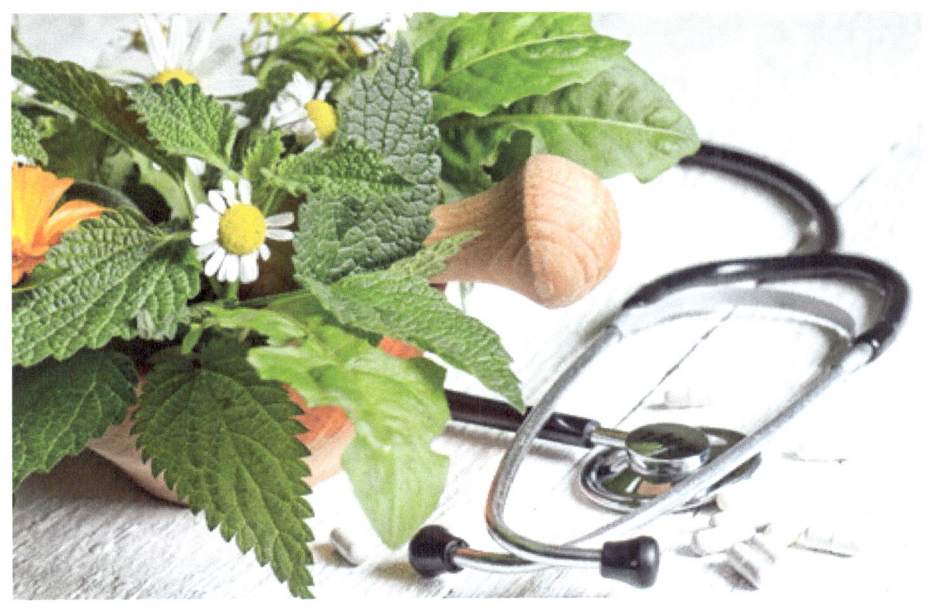

Back Cover Text

Integrative medical practitioners acknowledge links between body systems in treatment, recognize that illness and disease manifest uniquely in each patient, and address the complexity of each human being in an individualized manner. Fundamental concepts related to the Social Cognitive Theory (SCT) for understanding human behavior include outcome expectancy, self-efficacy, and skills. When working with targeted populations, public health practitioners can map-out the SCT to identify the social support, social network, and environmental factors affecting a community to achieve behavioral change. The SCT model can aid in the development of a plan of actions that public health practitioners can take next to address public health needs within a community in an integrative therapeutic manner.

Table of Contents

Integrative Healthcare	7
Social Cognitive Theory Key Features & Characteristics	11
SCT, Chronic Disease, & Self-Management Programs	14
Examples of Social Cognitive Theoretical Principles	14
Social Cognitive Theory Applied	16
Example of a Mapping Template using SCT	18
Influencing Actions of Chronically Ill Patients	29
Self-Regulation & Social Cognitive Theory	31
Conducting a Health Needs Assessment	35
Health Belief Model Case Study	47
Issue, Key Constructs, & Context of the Problem	49
Key Facts, Available Alternatives, & Recommendations	53
Integrative Medicine Research Journal Analysis	55
Integrative Healthcare Research	65
About the Author	71
Contact	72
Appendix	73
References	77

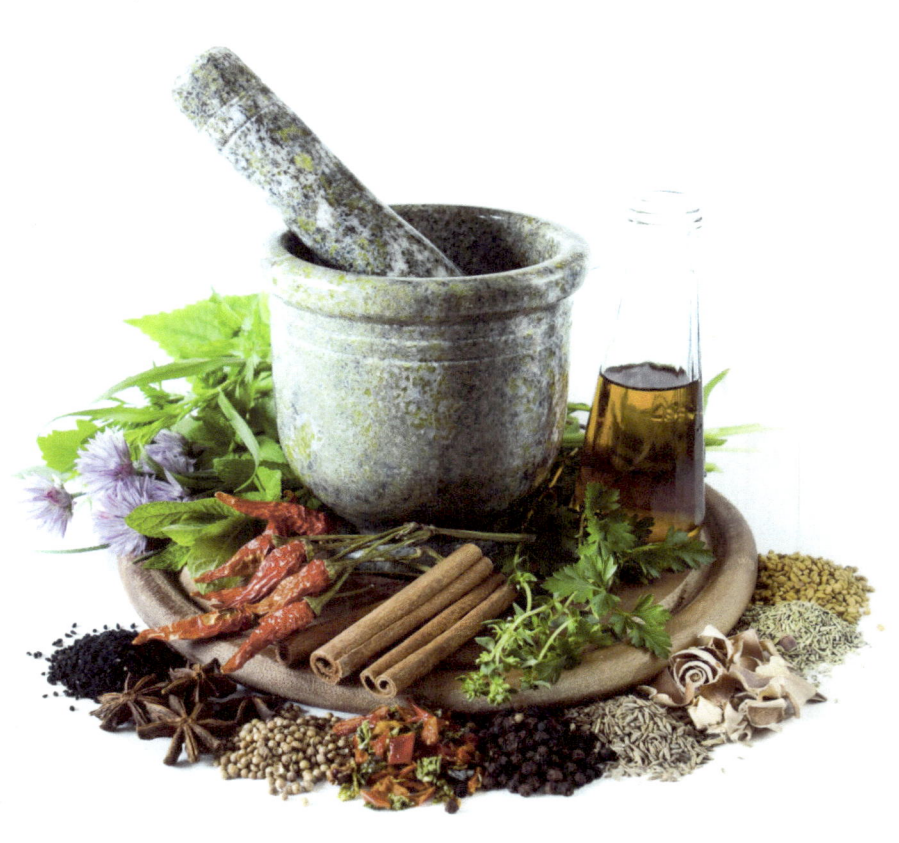

Integrative Healthcare

Integrative healthcare is as a comprehensive approach to medicine and general health and wellbeing that allows patients to be in the center of all care options and processes available from a natural holistic perspective (Ali & Katz, 2015; Witt, 2017). Rather than using one model of medical practice, the notion of integrative health can blend:

- complementary medicine,
- alternative care,
- Western herbalism,
- Eastern medicine,
- traditional naturopathy,
- functional medicine,
- Traditional Chinese Medicine, and
- homeopathy medicine to produce the most advantageous results for patients (Ang, Lee, Choi, Zhang, & Lee, 2020; Ang, Lee, Kim, Lee, & Lee, 2020; Chu, Sun, Huang, & Zhang, 2020; Ho, Chan, Chung, & Leung, 2020).

As reported by The Institute for Integrative Health (TIIH), the notion of integrative health is a condition of wellbeing in spirit, body, and mind reflecting the population, community, and individual (Witt, 2017). Satisfaction in healthcare can improve when the overall wellbeing of an individual is treated (Witt, 2017). When working from an integrative model, healthcare practitioners collaborate in a participatory manner, rather than separately in silos, to focus on all variables of a care plan delivered to a patient.

Doctors of reflexology, chiropractic care, biofeedback, acupressure, acupuncture, naturopathy, homeopath, western herbalism, Traditional Chinese Medicine, and eastern medicine are examples of alternative medicine (Chu, et al., 2020; Ho, et al., 2020; Witt, 2017). Health practitioners such as registered nurses, physical therapists, doctors of osteopath, and medical doctors are examples of conventional medicine. Integrative healthcare is a model that combines alternative or non-mainstream practices with conventional medicine commonly utilized in the western world (Khorsan, 2017; Witt, 2017). An alternative medicine approach to care can be described as using non-mainstream medicine in place of conventional medicine (Khorsan, 2017; Witt, 2017).

Thirty percent of Americans have admitted to utilizing products that are natural for medicinal treatments such as probiotics or herbs when treating ailments (RegisteredNursing.org, 2020). For example, when a patient synthesizes a medical care model that is integrated, he or she may include a doctor of osteopath and an acupuncturist for back pain (RegisteredNursing.org, 2020). A cancer patient may use conventional health insurance for various medical tests that are paid for such as blood work and then send results to a naturopathy doctor for vitamin C or hydrogen peroxide intravenous (IV) treatments that are not paid for by conventional health insurance.

Women who are pregnant may have an obstetrician who recommends western or eastern herbalism remedies for various common conditions during pregnancy rather than harmful pharmaceutical drugs that could damage the unborn child and the mother. One can research to find various medical practices throughout the country that specialize in an integrative care model utilizing a diversity of non-conventional and conventional specialists within the same practice (RegisteredNursing.org, 2020).

Despite how a conventional medical practitioner may feel about non-conventional medicine, one should be knowledgeable about an integrative healthcare model to educate patients, target populations, the overall public, and communities regarding healthcare options available (RegisteredNursing.org, 2020). Choices for healthcare should be considered for any medical condition, healthcare plan, and health insurance coverage.

Integrative Healthcare - Holistic Natural Medicine Model

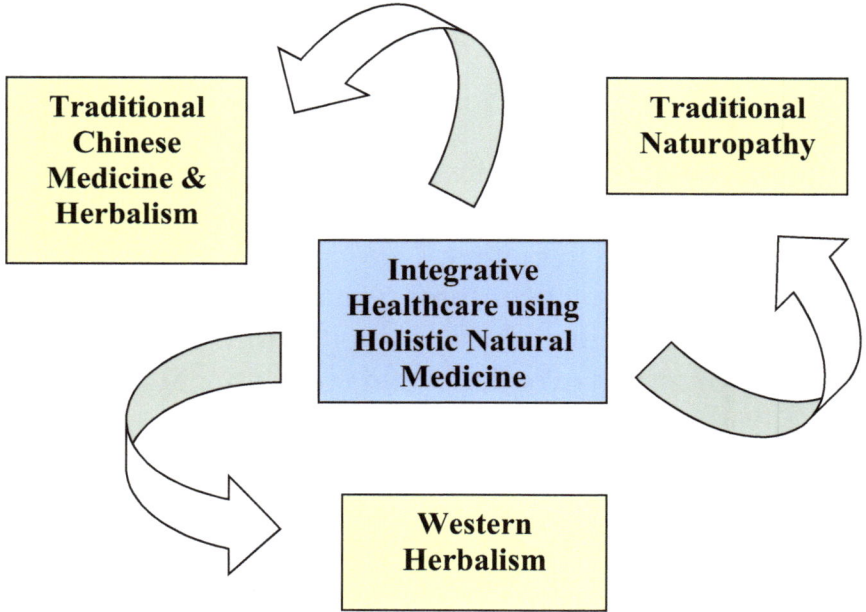

Adapted from Integrative Health Practitioner. (2019). *The 7 integrative disciplines of IHP*.

Social Cognitive Theory Key Features & Characteristics

This discussion will assess one peer-reviewed study using Social Cognitive Theory and key features and characteristics of the model. Examples of theoretical principles, models, constructs, and concepts used in the study are discussed. Finally, a case study scenario using the Social Cognitive Theory in application is presented. Bandura's Social Cognitive Theory graphic in Appendix.

Fundamental concepts related to the Social Cognitive Theory (SCT) for understanding human behavior include outcome expectancy, self-efficacy, and skills (Bandura, 1998; Bandura, 2004; LaMorte, 2016; Schunk & DiBenedetto, 2020; Sell, Amella, Mueller, Andrews, & Wachs, 2016). The principal concepts expressed within the theory relate to changing behavior and the capability of controlling one's own behavior. Social support systems, social networks, and the environment influence human behaviors. SCT is an adaptation of the Social Learning Theory and is formed on the notion that individuals acquire new knowledge by observing others (Bandura, 1998; Bandura, 2004; LaMorte, 2016).

The model posits that the behavior of humans is affected by on-going reciprocity between environmental, behavioral, and personal factors (Bandura, 1998; Bandura, 2004; LaMorte, 2016). SCT focuses on an individual's potential to change his or her environment to support the purposes one may devise for himself or herself (Schunk & DiBenedetto, 2020; Sell et al., 2016). For example, an individual can change his or her surroundings to meet one's desires. SCT indicates that shared activity throughout groups, such as organizations and social systems, is involved in the accomplishment of producing a change in the environment (Sell et al., 2016). Components of SCT encompass the following key aspects:

- "Reciprocal determinism,
- Outcome expectancy,
- Self-efficacy,
- Collective-efficacy,
- Observational learning,
- Incentive motivation,
- Facilitation,
- Self-regulation, and
- Moral disengagement" (Bandura, 1998; Bandura, 2004; LaMorte, 2016; Schunk & DiBenedetto, 2020; Sell et al., 2016).

When working with targeted populations, health educators can map-out the SCT to identify the social support, social network, and environmental factors affecting a community to achieve behavioral change (Bandura, 1998; Bandura, 2004; LaMorte, 2016; Sell et al., 2016). The SCT scenario-mapping template can aid in the development of a plan of actions health educators can take next to address public health needs within a community.

SCT, Chronic Disease, & Self-Management Programs

In a study conducted by Sell, Amella, Mueller, Andrews, and Wachs (2016), the SCT model was abstracted in an integrative review to examine primary scientific studies relating to chronic disease self-management in aging populations. The researchers found multiple gaps in the literature. Gaps included studies specifically targeting older adults, for example, adults over 65 with chronic disease, could not be obtained through the initial search parameters (Sell et al., 2016). A second search did not reveal sufficient results for inclusion criteria when searching for 60 years and older (Sell et al., 2016).

A tertiary search was conducted with 55 years and older to seek studies for inclusion in the integrative review (Sell et al., 2016). An additional limitation for inclusion in the integrative review included limited studies conducted over the last 10 years that reduced the sample size (Sell et al., 2016). Because a clear lack of research was evident with an older population experiencing chronic disease and self-management programs, the researchers sought to investigate the state of self-management and chronic disease applying to aging populations (Sell et al., 2016).

Furthermore, literature gaps revealed two other significant areas such as the impact of moral disengagement and self-management involving the use of social support (Sell et al., 2016). The researchers suggested that future studies should examine interventional and effectual long-term approaches addressing self-management success for aging populations (Sell et al., 2016). Unpublished studies such as manuscripts, conference proceedings, and dissertations were not included because empirical data was lacking relating to self-management program implementation (Sell et al., 2016).

Examples of Social Cognitive Theoretical Principles, Models, Constructs, & Concepts

According to Bandura (1998; 2004), SCT contributes both principles and predictors regarding how to motivate, guide, enable, and inform individuals to adopt habits promoting health and reducing behaviors impairing it. The model presents a mechanism for behavioral change that recognizes potential barriers and facilitators to success. The mechanism involves moderators such as the presence and quality of social influences, symbiotic relationships between individuals and the environment, and self-efficacy levels (Bandura, 1998; Bandura, 2004; Sell et al., 2016).

The SCT model involves comprehensive factors affecting the ability of individuals to change behaviors such as beliefs regarding behavioral change, successful self-management barriers, and goal setting (Bandura, 1998; Bandura, 2004; Sell et al., 2016). When health educators seek to aid individuals in changing negative behaviors, significant concepts such as moral disengagement, facilitation, incentive motivation, observational learning, outcome expectations, and reciprocal determinism can be integrated into public health education prevention and intervention programs (Bandura, 1998; Bandura, 2004; Sell et al., 2016). The integrative review categorized five domains, which included:

- Outcomes and self-efficacy linked to psychological determinants of behavior,
- Role modeling and motivation used in learning through observation,
- Interactions of the individual, society, and environment affecting environmental determinants of behavior,
- Self-monitoring aided by self-regulation,
- Feedback,
- Setting goals, and
- Moral disengagement whereby an individual's perception regarding existing behaviors may be altered via a change process (Sell et al., 2016).

Sell, Amella, Mueller, Andrews, and Wachs (2016), evaluated relevant studies that used these foundational concepts to identify gaps in self-management literature incorporating SCT domains to determine if inclusion in future research could enhance self-management.

Social Cognitive Theory Applied

The Social Cognitive Theory model can aid in development of comprehensive educational and behavior modification health programs for the public (Sell et al., 2016). Action plans for groups and individuals can be designed to assist the public in any type of health and wellness initiative, agenda, program, or curriculum model. The SCT model can aid health advocates when educating the public regarding the prevention of illness and the promotion of health via an integrative, naturopathy, holistic medicine perspective (Bandura, 1998; Bandura, 2004; LaMorte, 2016; Sell et al., 2016).

Furthermore, the theory can aid in the creation of differentiated and individualized health education messages to help the public make better health choices in daily life (Tomlinson, 2017; van Geel, Keuning, Frèrejean, Dolmans, van Merriënboer, & Visscher, 2019; Whitley, Gooderham, Duquette, Orders, & Cousins, 2019). The application of SCT can direct substantive educational tools and strategies for online instructional modules or in-person clinical visits with health providers and practioners.

A holistic, qualitative method can aid when addressing targeted individuals, groups, ability levels, cultural background, and specific health challenges. Moreover, cognitive dissonance theory should be considered when designing public health messages to address a lifetime of false and inaccurate information that has been disseminated to the public regarding health (Acharya, Blackwell, & Sen, 2018; Harmon-Jones, 2012).

The key is to work with the public in an individualized, holistic, naturopathy, integrative medicine model versus a one-size-fits-all, prescription-driven, allopathic, pharmaceutical system. Both the integrative medicine model and the manner of differentiating health instruction can be directed by individualized, holistic practices that effectively match the needs of targeted populations (Tomlinson, 2017; van Geel et al., 2019; Whitley et al., 2019).

The objective is to foster lifelong healthy habits, change negative behaviors, educate, inform, self-empower, and teach self-advocacy skills to the public regarding health and wellness (Bandura, 1998; Bandura, 2004; LaMorte, 2016; Schunk & DiBenedetto, 2020). Health educators can build a compare and contrast informational grid examining integrative medicine versus the allopathic system to assist the public in understanding what services are available and when, how, why, and who to use. A holistic, integrative instructional approach can be used to design curriculum to raise healthcare awareness in an intuitive, interactive, scaffolding, differentiated model that addresses learning styles, ability levels, and scaffolding techniques (Tomlinson, 2017; van Geel et al., 2019; Whitley et al., 2019).

Example of a Mapping Template using SCT

SCT components are applicable in changing health choices by evaluating health challenges of targeted populations in communities, countries, or regions. Pedagogical, interactive, intuitive, technology tools can be developed in various languages after curriculum is fully written. Public health education programs can be guided in clinics or in-person through workshops or can be accessible in an online manner.

The example presented explains how to map-out a health education agenda for the public regarding: (1) in-home self-care, (2) preventative healthcare, (3) natural diet, (4) natural remedies and products, and (5) integrative medicine services, providers, and doctors for healthcare needs.

Constructing	Defining	Case Study Scenario	Next Actions Health Educators can Take
Reciprocal Determinism	How environment can affect. How individuals can affect.	Target population feels they do not have the time to participate in a health education program or agenda. Address the environment. Address the people influencing the environment.	Present to the target population how to change the environment and/or the people so that they will have time to engage in a healthcare education agenda (Schunk & DiBenedetto, 2020). Address scheduling, time allotment, and time commitment issues.
Outcome Expectancy	The beliefs regarding the value and likelihood of ramifications related to behavioral	Address the target population's ability and desire to change the environment to enable	Evaluate whether target population feels they could possibly make alterations to

	decisions.	healthcare education.	their environment aiding them in health education pursuits (Sell et al., 2016). Evaluate if target population may place some value on health ramifications related to behavioral decisions (Sell et al., 2016).
Self-Efficacy	The beliefs regarding the capability to accomplish actions bringing about outcomes that are desired.	The target population believes they have the ability to make change happen.	Evaluate if target population is confident regarding choosing to make changes in one's schedule to participate in health educational pursuits (Sell et al., 2016). Aid in

			promoting the target population's comprehension regarding where and how to seek out accurate and credible health-related information and scientific facts over fake news.
Efficacy of Collective	The assumptions about the capability of a targeted community to accomplish cooperative behaviors bringing about outcomes that are desired.	The target population can form social networks such as communities, churches, schools, neighborhoods, and groups.

Social networks can include websites, social media sites, email, and other Internet modalities connecting individuals and groups globally. | Examine the target population's social structure to assess individuals that may be supporting of positive changes in lifestyle to address health issues (Bandura, 1998; Bandura, 2004; Sell et al., 2016).

Social systems |

			where "buddies" can be established are advantageous in assisting in accountability to others in the group or community (Bandura, 1998; Bandura, 2004; Sell et al., 2016).

Relevant, current sharing and learning assists the movement toward changing behaviors. |
| **Observational Learning** | Learn to accomplish different behavior via peer-modeling, interpersonal interactions, or exposure to displays of these factors | Target populations can learn health promotion techniques, practice conscientious outcomes, and make achievable targets to | Create and facilitate online and in-person discussion groups, seminars, and curriculum modules to aid the target population in |

22

	in media or educational experiences.	address a deficit in healthcare awareness.	reaching manageable objectives. Determine doable outcomes (Bandura, 1998; Bandura, 2004; Sell et al., 2016). Accommodate and modify strategies to overcome barriers and foster growth (Bandura, 1998; Bandura, 2004; Sell et al., 2016).
Incentive Motivation	The misuse or use of punishments or rewards to change behavior.	Evaluate motivational strategies for target populations to pursue health education (Schunk & DiBenedetto, 2020). Evaluate	Categorize de-motivation and motivation factors (Bandura, 1998; Bandura, 2004; Schunk & DiBenedetto, 2020; Sell et

		significant barriers hindering participation, commitment, and self-motivation in educational pursuits (Schunk & DiBenedetto, 2020).	al., 2016).
Facilitation	How to provide environmental changes, resources, or tools to aid in making new behaviors less difficult to do.	Specific examples could be: calendar planning to engage in self-education pursuits, scheduling, and journaling (Schunk & DiBenedetto, 2020). Foster examples of family, parent, group, and peer successes.	Administer to the target population the needed resources and tools to help them become more able to participate in health educational pursuits (Bandura, 1998; Bandura, 2004; Sell et al., 2016).
Self-Regulation	How to control self via social support enlistment, self-	Target population can manage their schedule independently and organize	Describe the components designed in a health education model to aid

	instruction, self-reward, feedback, goal setting, and self-monitoring.	educational pursuits. Individuals can manage their own schedule to meet achievable goals, self-monitor, and self-education pursuits (Schunk & DiBenedetto, 2020). Pedagogical systems can design-in assessment, monitors, and time management tools.	the target population in accomplishing self-education, self-awareness, and self regulation (Schunk & DiBenedetto, 2020). Pedagogical lessons can be designed to track participation, track performance, be easy-to-use, intuitive, and monitor various educational milestones.
Moral Disengagement	How individuals think regarding behaviors that are harmful. Why suffering can be viewed as acceptable	Not engaging in self-education pursuits, can lead to unhealthy decisions. Misguided information from inaccurate	Evaluate other factors, variables, tools, institutions, groups, organizations partnerships, and individuals

	when inflicted on self or others.	and false authority can have harmful effects on public health.

False information regarding healthcare is harmful and damaging to the public. Inaccurate information fosters similar negative behavioral choices made by others within the target population. An incompetence to self-educate is harmful to others in the family. | that may be useful in promoting the health agenda and lowering negative aspects of limited health awareness and knowledge (Bandura, 1998; Bandura, 2004; Sell et al., 2016).

Advance and foster health education, information, trusted news sources, and resources for the entire community.

Describe and teach strategies to the target population so that they can empower others within their sphere of influence |

| | | | (Bandura, 1998; Bandura, 2004; Schunk & DiBenedetto, 2020; Sell et al., 2016). |

An SCT educational health plan can address health behaviors to aid target populations in making behavior modifications by:

1. Providing on-going educational tools,
2. Providing touch-base, check-in, and follow-up services,
3. Providing access to support groups,
4. Supporting with alternatives, providers, services, and multiple resources,
5. Informing with accurate health news and information, and
6. Educating with comprehensive and differentiated tools servicing needs of the community (Bandura, 1998; Bandura, 2004; LaMorte, 2016; Sell et al., 2016).

An SCT mapping template can provide the mapping-out or overall vision of public health educational objectives and goals targeting specific populations. Public health education plans are further developed in the design of curriculum and messaging applying directly to the health concerns of a community. The health education plan should include differentiated program development tools, providers, services, workshops, instructional modules, techniques, strategies, objectives, goals, principals, and theories described with greater depth and detail (Tomlinson, 2017; van Geel et al., 2019; Whitley et al., 2019).

Conclusion

This discussion assessed one peer-reviewed study using Social Cognitive Theory and key features and characteristics of the model. Examples of theoretical principles, models, constructs, and concepts used in the study were discussed. Finally, a case study scenario using the Social Cognitive Theory in application was presented. Bandura's Social Cognitive Theory graphic in Appendix.

Influencing Actions of Chronically Ill Patients with Social Cognitive Theory

The discussion examines how Social Cognitive Theory (SCT) can influence the behaviors and actions of chronically ill patients. The theory's constructions are identified in a table. Two published health articles are compared to the theory's tenets and constructs.

The discussion focuses on the Belil, Alhani, Ebadi, and Kazemnejad (2018) study and an interventional plan is presented with each of the 11 SCT domains. The discussion develops an intervention for each of the constructs missing from the study. Additional research regarding Social Cognitive Theory (SCT) constructs and how the categories can be used in a healthcare setting are presented. Each construct category is addressed to explain how a health intervention can be implemented. Three Social Cognitive Theory graphics are located in the Appendix to support the discussion.

Self-Efficacy & Social Cognitive Theory

Belil, Alhani, Ebadi, and Kazemnejad (2018)

In a study conducted by Belil et al. (2018), various aspect of self-efficacy were explored in patients experiencing chronic physical conditions. The qualitative study was conducted in two university hospitals with 22 participants that included nurses, family caregivers, and patients who were chronically ill (Belil et al., 2018). Data collection was coded and themed into 247 analysis units over eight subcategories with 4 generic categories. The findings identified various aspects of self-efficacy in chronically ill patients that may be utilized to establish and actualize programs to aid in empowering others with similar health challenges (Belil et al., 2018).

Examples of categories identified in the coded and themed analysis included adjusting interpersonal relationships, performing self-care activities, planning for life, and management of emotions (Belil et al., 2018). The study findings indicated that the self-efficacy of chronic patients consisted of social, functional, psycho-emotional, and cognitive categories that can be utilized to evaluate empowerment (Belil et al., 2018). Furthermore, the identification of dimensions can aid in a holistic assessment of self-efficacy levels in patients (Belil et al., 2018).

The researchers posited that these findings can be used as a baseline for designing effective health interventions to increase empowerment and self-efficacy in patients with chronic illness (Belil et al., 2018). The findings can significantly aid in addressing the development of strengthening social relationships, improving stress management and emotions, enhancing caring performance, and developing personal knowledge in chronically ill patients (Belil et al., 2018).

Self-Regulation & Social Cognitive Theory

Tougas, Hayden, McGrath, Huguet, and Rozario (2015)

In a systematic review conducted by Tougas, Hayden, McGrath, Huguet, and Rozario (2015), the extent that theory is established and integrated into existing interventions was examined. Multiple databases were searched such as EMBASE, CENTRAL, PsycINFO, and PubMed up to May 2014. In addition, citations were searched in Web of Science, lists of references of systematic studies and reviews, and registered protocols in clinicaltrials.gov were included in the search parameters.

Moreover, peer-reviewed studies documenting interventions referencing self-regulation themes related to Social Cognitive Theory and managing chronic health illnesses were included (Tougas et al., 2015). The systematic review findings narrowed down 35 intervention studies that documented self-regulation and self-monitoring components in the Social Cognitive Theory model. Of the 35 studies that were included, 21 adequately integrated characteristics addressing each of the Social Cognitive Theory components. The intervention studies included self-evaluation, self-judgment, and self-monitoring instruments (Tougas et al., 2015).

Examples of construct categories identified included external rewards, self-incentives, and feedback and consistency (Tougas et al., 2015). The researchers established that a systematic review is an effective tool for identifying the self-regulation component of Social Cognitive Theory. Finally, the theory is a useful framework for guiding the intervention development for chronically ill patients.

Social Cognitive Theory Constructs

Identified Constructs of Social Cognitive Theory	Belil et al. (2018) Self-Efficacy and SCT	Tougas et al. (2015) Self-Regulation and SCT
"Facilitation and Behavioral Capability		
Reciprocal Determinism		
Emotional Coping Responses		
Outcome Expectations		
Self-Efficacy	Self-efficacy was explored in chronically ill patients in the SCT model (Belil et al., 2018).	
Collective Efficacy		
Observational Learning		
Incentive Motivation		
Self-Regulation (Self-Control)		Self-evaluation, self-judgment, and self-monitoring was examined in chronically ill patients in the self-regulation

		category of SCT (Tougas et al., 2015).
Moral Disengagement"		

Conducting a Health Needs Assessment for Chronically Ill Patients using Social Cognitive Theory

This section focuses on the Belil et al. (2018) study previously examined. The discussion develops an intervention for each of the constructs missing from the study. Additional research regarding Social Cognitive Theory (SCT) constructs and how the categories can be used in a healthcare setting are presented. Each construct category is addressed to explain how a health intervention can be implemented. The study findings in Belil et al. (2018) represented various SCT self-efficacy aspects exhibited by chronically ill patients that can be further developed and implemented in empowerment programs for the chronically ill.

Belil et al. (2018) Self-Efficacy Findings

The direction of the Belil et al. (2018) study was to understand and develop self-efficacy in chronically ill patients. Efficacy of self is a multi-dimensional concept. For the empowerment process, the concept can be understood in terms of acquired skills, predisposing factors, and the empowerment index (Belil et al., 2018). The study findings indicated that self-efficacy is the capability of patients to develop understanding and knowledge in relationship to self-care and illness via non-virtual and virtual scientific and personal resources (Belil et al., 2018).

Furthermore, the findings indicated that self-efficacy is about managing one's excitement in ways that permit patients to continue living with self-care and illness, lifestyle planning, maintaining job performance, and establishing daily relationships with others (Belil et al., 2018). The self-efficacy dimensions documented in the study included social, functional, psycho-emotional, and cognitive (Belil et al., 2018).

The chronically ill participants in the study used the self-efficacy dimensions to resourcefully seek and find solutions for illness-related issues, obtain sufficient knowledge about afflictions and therapeutics, manage and control psycho-emotional life processes, and develop positive interpersonal relationships (Belil et al., 2018).

Intervention Development

Since the Belil et al. (2018) study only addressed one category of the 11 SCT domains; the other 10 will be addressed in this intervention plan for chronically ill patients. The intervention plan can be used in any healthcare setting with patients or clients needing help with chronic illness. Significant constructs of SCT that are important to intervention plans include self-efficacy, self-control, reinforcement, and observational learning (Bandura, 1998; Bandura, 2004; LaMorte, 2016). Behavior modification principles typically used to foster change are derived from SCT. Various factors of behavioral interventions such as reinforcement, efficacy of self, and control of self involve monitoring of self, behavioral contracting, and goal setting (McAlister, Perry, & Parcel, 2008; Schunk & DiBenedetto, 2020).

Self-efficacy is an individual's belief in his or her capability in making progress toward a goal and enduring in the actions required in spite of challenges and obstacles (Bandura, 1998; Bandura, 2004; LaMorte, 2016). This SCT domain appears to be particularly important for affecting healthy behavioral changes. Health practitioners can make intentional efforts to aid in the development of self-efficacy in patients by applying three specific techniques such as:

- Setting achievable, incremental, and small goals;
- Assigning formal behavioral contracting to create objectives and determine rewards; and
- Monitor and reinforce, along with self-monitoring tasks by patients maintaining records (Bandura, 1998; Bandura, 2004; LaMorte, 2016; McAlister et al., 2008; Schunk & DiBenedetto, 2020).

In collective intervention programs involving nutrition, it can be beneficial to add activities such as self-monitoring, problem-solving discussions, and cooking demonstrations that are grounded in SCT constructs. The SCT construct of reciprocal determinism addresses a patient as a change agent and a change responder. Hence, reinforcements, role model examples, and changes in the environment can be promoted to foster healthy behavioral change (Bensley & Brookins-Fisher, 2019; Cottrell, Girvan, McKenzie, & Seabert, 2018).

Reciprocal Determinism

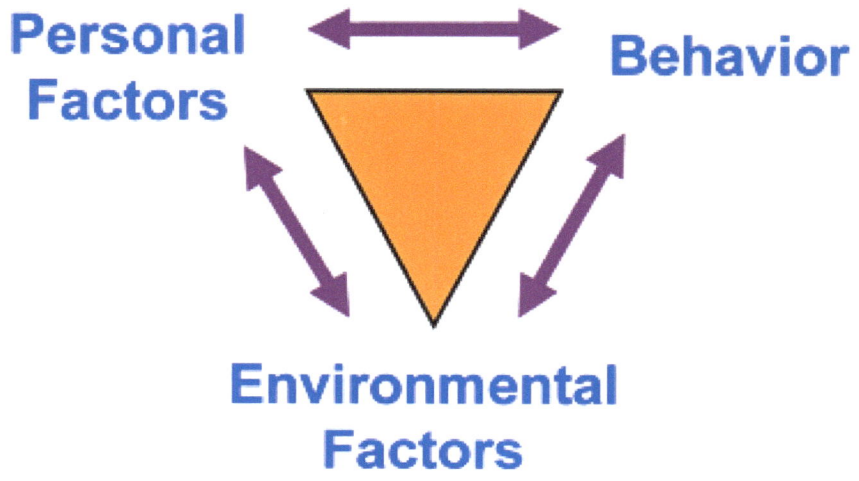

The SCT model in intervention plans focuses on dynamic interactions between individuals known as personal factors, their environments, and their behaviors (Bandura, 1998; Bandura, 2004; LaMorte, 2016). These factors continuously interact by affecting and being affected by each other. When including the reciprocal determinism domain in an intervention plan, consider various ways to foster behavioral change such as targeting attitudes and knowledge in addition to making environmental changes (Doyle, Ward, & Early, 2019; Glanz, Rimer, & Lewis, 2002).

A key concept regarding efficacy of self involves a patient's confidence in his or her ability to achieve certain behaviors when various challenges are presented.

Self-efficacy can be improved upon by using four distinct approaches: (1) experiences of personal success, (2) social modeling revealing how others in similar situations with similar characteristics have taken steps to achieve similar behavioral changes; (3) repairing emotional and physical conditions, and (4) verbal persuasion of others encouraging and boosting confidence (McAlister, Perry, & Parcel, 2008; Schunk & DiBenedetto, 2020).

In the observational learning domain, healthcare practioners can aid patients by providing credible role models reflecting the patient's target population who have mastered the desired behaviors (Bensley & Brookins-Fisher, 2019; Cottrell et al., 2018).

Furthermore, the SCT self-regulation domain can be realized using six distinct methods such as:

1. Systematic observation and self-monitoring of a patient's behavior of self;
2. Setting goals;
3. Feedback regarding performance quality and how improvements can be made;
4. Rewarding self;
5. Self-direction and instruction; and
6. Social supports from others encouraging a patient's attempts and achievements in exerting

self-control (Bandura, 1998; Bandura, 2004; LaMorte, 2016).

In addition, four distinct factors associated with supportive behaviors in the social support category can include the following aspects:

1. Appraisal supports such as useful information for the purposes of self-evaluation, for example, feedback that is constructive,
2. Informational supports such as information, suggestions, and advice that a patient can effectively utilize when addressing obstacles and problems,
3. Instrumental supports that include services, resources, and aid explicitly assisting a patient's needs, and
4. Emotional supports that include factors such as caring, trust, love, and empathy (McAlister et al., 2008; Schunk & DiBenedetto, 2020).

Moreover, intervention plans can use new technologies such as websites, Internet newsletters, video conferencing, podcasting, live streams, videos, social media, email communication, and online interactive curriculum modules to support application of SCT (Doyle et al., 2019; Glanz et al., 2002). In addition to addressing other aspects of the SCT model, new technologies can aid in fostering encouragement, constructive and supportive feedback, verbal persuasion, and modeling (Bensley & Brookins-Fisher, 2019; Cottrell et al., 2018).

The concept of outcome expectations involves the beliefs a patient has regarding value and likelihood of consequences related to behavioral choices. In this SCT domain, health practioners can aid patients by demonstrating positive outcomes that can occur when performing desired behaviors (Doyle et al., Glanz et al., 2002). The collective efficacy domain involves belief or confidence in a group's capability to bring about desired changes. In this SCT domain, health practioners can bring individuals together to compel a call to action.

Health educators can design activities, interactions, and fellowship opportunities for groups to feel connected and aid in advancing self-confidence in accomplishing desired behavioral changes (Bensley & Brookins-Fisher, 2019; Cottrell et al., 2018). In the facilitation and behavioral capability domain, health practitioners can aid in providing environmental changes, resources, and tools to patients to assist them in making new behaviors easier to accomplish (Doyle et al., 2019; Glanz et al., 2002). This can be done by providing patients with skills-based training as well as knowledge-based training in a comprehensive intervention program.

The incentive motivation domain involves the use of punishments and rewards to modify a patient's behaviors. Health practitioners can investigate what types of incentives may motivate patients to participate in an intervention program (Doyle et al., 2019; Glanz et al., 2002). The moral disengagement domain is about a lack of moral standards that involves how individuals think about harmful behaviors (Bandura, 1998; Bandura, 2004; LaMorte, 2016). In addition, this lack of moral standards can aid in making infliction of suffering acceptable when individuals disengaging from moral self-regulation.

Health educators can use this SCT domain by re-engaging self-regulatory moral standards in a way that illuminates potential diffusion and dehumanization of accountability onto others (McAlister et al., 2008; Schunk & DiBenedetto, 2020). Finally, yet extremely important, in the emotional coping responses domain, health educators can teach patients specific tactics and strategies to help them manage emotional stimuli (Bensley & Brookins-Fisher, 2019; Cottrell et al., 2018).

Constructs in Social Cognitive Theory

Social Cognitive Theory Constructs	Belil et al. (2018) Self-Efficacy and SCT	Behavioral Intervention Plan for Chronically Ill Patients
"Facilitation and Behavioral Capability		Provide environmental changes, resources, and tools to assist in making new behaviors easier to accomplish (Doyle et al., 2019; Glanz et al., 2002). Provide skills-based training and knowledge-based training.
Reciprocal Determinism		Reinforcements, role model examples, and changes in the environment promote healthy behavioral change (Bensley & Brookins-Fisher, 2019; Cottrell et al., 2018).
Emotional Coping Responses		Teach specific tactics and strategies to help manage emotional stimuli (Bensley & Brookins-Fisher, 2019; Cottrell et al., 2018).
Outcome Expectations		Demonstrate positive outcomes that can occur when performing desired behaviors (Doyle et al., Glanz et al., 2002).

Self-Efficacy	Understanding and knowledge in relationship to self-care and illness via non-virtual and virtual scientific and personal resources (Belil et al., 2018). Managing excitement to continue living with self-care and illness, lifestyle planning, maintaining job performance, and establishing daily relationships (Belil et al., 2018).	Make intentional efforts to aid in the development of self-efficacy by applying techniques such as setting achievable, incremental, and small goals, behavioral contracting, monitor, reinforce, and record-keeping (Bandura, 1998; Bandura, 2004; LaMorte, 2016; McAlister et al., 2008; Schunk & DiBenedetto, 2020).
Collective Efficacy		Bring individuals together to compel a call to action. Design activities,

		interactions, and fellowship opportunities for groups to feel connected. Aid in advancing self-confidence in accomplishing desired behavioral changes (Bensley & Brookins-Fisher, 2019; Cottrell et al., 2018).
Observational Learning		Provide credible role models reflecting the patient's target population who have mastered desired behaviors (Bensley & Brookins-Fisher, 2019; Cottrell et al., 2018).
Incentive Motivation		Investigate what types of incentives motivate patients to participate in an intervention program (Doyle et al., 2019; Glanz et al., 2002).
Self-Regulation (Self-Control)		Systematic observation and self-monitoring of a patient's behavior of self; Setting goals; Feedback regarding performance quality and how improvements can be made;

		Rewarding self; Self-direction and instruction; Social supports encouraging a patient's attempts and achievements in exerting self-control (Bandura, 1998; Bandura, 2004; LaMorte, 2016).
Moral Disengagement"		Re-engage self-regulatory moral standards to illuminate potential diffusion and dehumanization of accountability onto others (McAlister et al., 2008; Schunk & DiBenedetto, 2020). Teach specific tactics and strategies to help manage emotional stimuli (Bensley & Brookins-Fisher, 2019; Cottrell et al., 2018).

Conclusion

The discussion examined how Social Cognitive Theory can influence the behaviors and actions of chronically ill patients. The theory's constructs were identified in a table. Two published health articles were compared to the theory's tenets and constructs. In addition, the discussion focused on the Belil et al. (2018) study and an interventional plan was presented with each of the 11 SCT domains. The discussion developed an intervention for each of the constructs missing from the study. Additional research regarding Social Cognitive Theory (SCT) constructs and how the categories can be used in a healthcare setting were presented. Each construct category was addressed to explain how a health intervention could be implemented. Three Social Cognitive Theory graphics are located in the Appendix to support the discussion.

Health Belief Model Case Study

This discussion will analyze a Health Belief Model (HBM) case study. Factors such as issues involved, key constructs, context of the problem, key facts that should be considered, alternatives available to the decision-maker, and recommendations will be examined. With complimentary and alternative medicine (CAM) therapies and usage on the rise, Agunbiade (2019) sought to understand the phenomenon using the HBM.

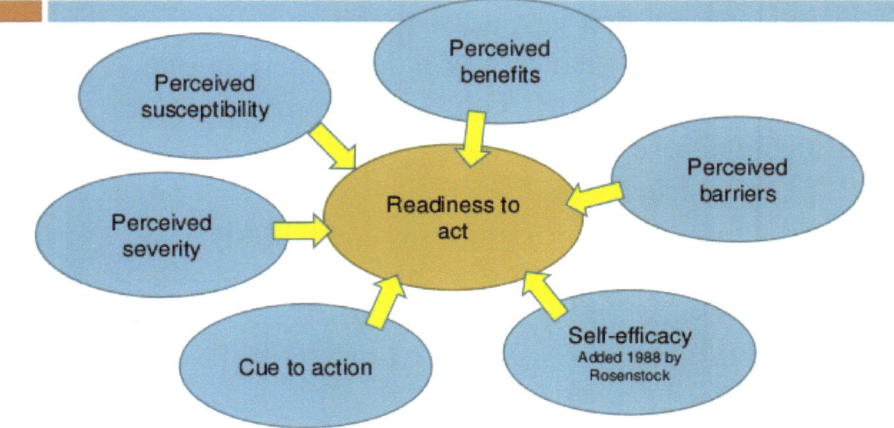

Adapted from Tan, C-E. (2014, October 11). *Health behaviour and health education for family medicine postgraduates.* https://www.slideshare.net/ChaiEngTan/health-behaviour-and-health-education-for-family-medicine-postgraduates-40155488

Issue, Key Constructs, & Context of the Problem

In a study conducted by Agunbiade (2019), the reasons for flourishing use of herbal medicine in New York City and how the use of the medicines are experienced is documented in a case study. The conceptual framework for the study involved the HBM. The HBM can be a basis for explaining factors influencing the decision-making process individuals engage in when embracing new forms of health solutions (Agunbiade, 2019).

HBM involves six variables, which include the following: (1) perceived severity, (2) perceived susceptibility, (3) perceived benefit, (4) perceived barriers, (5) cues to action, and (6) self-efficacy (Conley et al., 2018). The model was significant to the study to aid in explaining participant choices regarding medicine and the embracing of herbal medicine usage (Agunbiade, 2019; Conley et al., 2018). Furthermore, the model explained participants' understanding about conventional medicine and the rationale regarding a change to alternative forms of medicine (Agunbiade, 2019).

Data analysis consisted of personal context with reference to other data sources. Data triangulation consisted of comparing this study with several other research studies to confirm data from unrelated and broad measurement procedures (Agunbiade, 2019). Primary data was developed in the study from face-to-face interviews and secondary data involved a survey questionnaire and flyers from herbal stores, pamphlets, leaflets, brochures, herbal medicine practitioners' websites, and commercial billboards (Agunbiade, 2019).

According to Agunbiade (2019), noticeable gaps in the literature included conventional medicine treatment causing challenges to individuals suffering adverse reactions to pharmaceutical drugs and desiring gentler forms of medicine. Moreover, the researcher discovered an academic gap in the literature regarding the understanding of consequences related to herbal medicine usage (Agunbiade, 2019).

The researcher focused on studying the reasons for why New York Americans are choosing CAM and herbal medicine. Research to date on the topic focused on the efficacy, safety, and prevalence of herbal medicine use (Kennedy et al., 2016). With a rise in CAM and herbal medicine use, and a gap in the literature related to understanding the consequences of herbal medicine usage, a study about how CAM practitioners educate the public is warranted. The findings explained that medication side effects and family influence were contributing factors regarding the increased use of herbal and natural medicines.

Furthermore, the study findings were congruent with Chan, Tay, Shih, Tan, and Chiang (2012) and Kircher, Watson-Whitmyre, and Montvilo (2008) and further illustrated the severity of reactions participants experienced using conventional medicine and how changing to herbal medicine removed symptoms.

Key constructs of the study included ten New York Americans between 25 years and 65 years of age responding to open-ended interview questions and survey questionnaires (Agunbiade, 2019). Research indicates that many Americans suffer from various diseases, autoimmune problems, and chronic pain (Agunbiade, 2019; Mehl-Madova, Managuy, & Plummer, 2016; NIH, 2020).

Furthermore, many individuals suffering from chronic health challenges can have adverse reactions to conventional pharmaceutical drugs and allopathic treatments (Mehl-Madova, Managuy, & Plummer, 2016). In the 2018 National Institutes of Health (NIH) report, 128 individuals die everyday in the United States after an opioid overdose (NIH, 2020). The addiction and misuse of opioids, synthetic opioids such as fentanyl, and prescription pain relievers is a chronic epidemic affecting the economic and social welfare of public health (NIH, 2020). The Centers for Disease Control and Prevention reported that the overall burden to the economy related to the misuse of allopathic prescription opioids is $78.5 billion a year (NIH, 2020). In addition to exorbitant healthcare costs, other costs to public health include justice and criminal involvement, addiction treatment, and lost productivity (NIH, 2020).

Key Facts, Available Alternatives, & Recommendations

Complimentary and alternative medicine therapies can be used to provide effective pain management for individuals dealing with chronic pain challenges rather than pharmaceutical allopathic prescription opiates (Mehl-Madova, Managuy, & Plummer, 2016). The researcher designed a qualitative case study method to interview 10 participants regarding views about experiences transitioning from allopathic pharmaceutical prescription drugs to the use of CAM. Qualitative open-ended interview questions were design in addition to a survey questionnaire to examine the reasons for increased use of CAM and why and how participants embraced the use of herbal medicine.

A case study design was appropriate for this study to examine behaviors of the group as a whole. A quantitative design would not provide a rich, deep, and wide range of expression that captures individualized and group experiences related to CAM usage, beliefs, rationale, and the effects experienced by the participants involved in the study.

Alternatives the researcher could consider might be a different type of design involving more participants such as 15 to 20 and do a phenomenology approach for this topic. A quantitative study is not appropriate for this topic because others interested in this area want to hear and comprehend the voice of participants and the decisions made regarding CAM use versus manufactured pharmaceutical drugs. Recommendations for further research can involve why individuals from a variety of socioeconomic and cultural backgrounds choose CAM remedies and therapeutics over pharmaceuticals. In addition, future quantitative research can measure patient satisfaction and disatisfaction with CAM versus pharmaceuticals.

Conclusion

This discussion analyzed a Health Belief Model (HBM) case study. Factors such as issues involved, key constructs, context of the problem, key facts that should be considered, alternatives available to the decision-maker, and recommendations were examined. With complimentary and alternative medicine (CAM) therapies and usage on the rise, Agunbiade (2019) explained the phenomenon using the HBM.

Integrative Medicine Research Journal Analysis

This discussion analyzes four journal articles published in Integrative Medicine Research, volume 10, issue 1, March 2021. The discussion analyzes three systematic reviews and one qualitative design. In addition, one dissertation study is summarized regarding multiple aspects supporting fundamental conditions of an efficacious integrative healthcare model in the United States.

Ng, Nault, & Nazir (2021)

In a study conducted by Ng, Nault, and Nazir (2021), clinical practice guidelines (CPGs) describing quality and quantity of lung cancer recommendations containing complementary and integrative medicine (CIM) identified that only a limited amount CPGs are available to aid substantive and knowledgeable decision-making between health care practitioners and patients with regard to CIM therapeutics. The study involved a systematic review identifying CPGs for lung cancer. Databases such as CINAHL, EMBASE, and MEDLINE were explored between 2008 through 2018 (Ng et al., 2021).

In addition, websites such as the National Center for Complementary and Integrative Health and the Guidelines International Network were searched (Ng et al., 2021). Finally, guidelines eligible for the study included lung cancer recommendations for management and treatment. The guidelines were evaluated using the Research and Evaluation II (AGREE II) instrument – Guidelines Appraisal (Ng et al., 2021).

CIM is broadly sought out by cancer patients (Ng et al., 2021). Up to 50% of patients with lung cancer in the United States seek these therapies (Ng et al., 2021). Of 589 different search results, CIM was mentioned by four guidelines. Three of those four guidelines made recommendations for CIM. Measured percentages by domain from lowest to highest included the following categories: (1) applicability, (2) stakeholder involvement, (3) rigor of development, (4) editorial independence, (5) clarity and presentation, and (6) scope and purpose (Ng et al., 2021). Merely one CPG was identified for providing a comprehensive recommendations list for CIM. The researchers stated that a range of various factors can be attributed to this finding, although it is likely that an absence of quality controlled and randomized research on CIM therapies can be attributed (Ng et al., 2021).

Additional variables challenging complementary and integrative medicine research involve an absence of CIM practitioner research training. Furthermore, a lack of funding and resources to advance CIM training and expertise, researcher bias against using complementary and integrative medicine, and an absence of comprehensive CIM training and knowledge across medical disciplines, present additional challenges (Ng et al., 2021). Based upon increased public interest to use CIM therapies and remedies, the researchers believe it is important for rigorous and continued research to develop in this area of medicine.

Findings and recommendations in the study indicated various and multiple assessment tools, criteria, checklists, frameworks, and principles available to CPG creators to produce quality CPGs relevant to complementary and integrative medicine therapeutics (Ng et al., 2021). In addition, researcher findings and recommendations explained that guidelines measuring well in the study could provide a framework for conversations amongst healthcare practitioners and patients involving the use of CIM therapeutics regarding lung cancer. Lower measured guidelines identified in the study could be enhanced by utilizing the AGREE II instrument with additional guideline development resources (Ng et al., 2021).

Chunga, Wong, Zhong, Tjioe, Leung, & Griffiths (2021)

In a systematic review study conducted by Chunga, Wong, Zhong, Tjioe, Leung, and Griffiths (2021), sources such as the Cochrane Complementary Medicine website was searched for clinical evidence supporting the use of traditional and complementary medicine (TCM). Furthermore, full reports and synopses for the Regional Strategy for Traditional Medicine in the Western Pacific 2011–2020 and the WHO Traditional Medicine Strategy 2014–2023 were examined in the study (Chunga et al., 2021; WHO, 2012; WHO, 2013). In addition, additional methods identified in the study included publications searched in MEDLINE from inception through 2020, April (Chunga et al., 2021). The researchers focused on studies regarding how older individuals perceive TCM. Policies for the integration of TCM into health models using analysis from patient choice and current evidence-based studies were recommended.

Researchers concluded that a train the trainer approach would be an effective and efficient method of promoting and maximizing self-care modalities using evidence-based TCM (Chunga et al., 2021). Findings included experiences throughout multiple countries and various income levels. Results represented a popularity of natural products. Researchers recommended that policy makers establish pharmacovigilance detection for the possibility of harm, implementing quality assurance, and guiding the appropriate regulation of natural products (Chunga et al., 2021).

Additionally, pharmacists' role when consulting with individuals regarding the use of natural remedies and self-medication should be strengthened (Chunga et al., 2021). Finally, recommendations for cooperative regulatory frameworks at global and regional levels for natural products could be beneficial to the public. Researchers noted that patient protection, improved standards, and mutual understanding of regulatory approval could be a priority in medicine and healthcare models (Chunga et al., 2021). The researchers believe the promotion of healthy aging throughout the course of life should be a priority in medicine models. Because TCM is popular in the Western Pacific Region, possibilities regarding exploring the use and application of TCM for healthy aging should be considered in policy development.

Gerontakos, Casteleijn, & Wardlea (2021)

In a study conducted by Gerontakos, Casteleijn, and Wardlea (2021), suggestions for further examination of practitioner knowledge derived from clinical experience and intuition could aid in specifying codification of core clinical concepts, standardization, and additional clarity typically used by Chinese Medicine (CM) practitioners. These types of coding and classifications have been absent in scientific and biomedical literature descriptions. The qualitative study used thematic analysis and focus groups with naturopaths in Australia to measure adaptogenic use and application outcomes expected by the practitioners when working with patients.

Seventeen naturopaths with over five years clinical experience with bachelor degrees and higher were involved in three focus groups. Main themes identified in the study included: (1) intersystem activity, (2) having a restorative effect, (3) raising vitality, (4) divergent perceptions regarding knowledge sources about adaptogens, and (5) ambiguous cultural origins of adaptogens (Gerontakos et al., 2021). Additional sub-themes were identified.

According to the researchers, the concept of adaptogens seems to align well with the lexicon of naturopathic principles. The use and application of adaptogen remedies match well with fundamental precepts of naturopathic practice such as: (1) the concept of treating the whole person, (2) restoring harmony, and (3) raising vitality (Gerontakos et al., 2021). The principle of naturopathic medicine refers to the notion of treating the whole person using an individualized medicine approach.

Naturopathic practitioners: (1) acknowledge links between body systems in treatment, (2) recognize that illness and disease manifest uniquely in each patient, and (3) address the complexity of each human being in an individualized manner (Gerontakos et al., 2021). Adaptogens were perceived as medicines by the naturopaths as having cohesive alignment with naturopathic principles. Furthermore, adaptogens were perceived to have the ability to holistically restore homeostasis throughout numerous systems within the body when practitioners selected certain adaptogens based upon a patient's individualized presentation (Gerontakos et al., 2021).

Iranzadasl, Karimi, Moadeli, & Pasalar (2021)

In a study conducted by Iranzadasl, Karimi, Moadeli, and Pasalar (2021), a narrative systematic review analyzed authoritative Persian medicine books that were published from the 9th and 19th centuries AD. In addition, medical databases such as Google Scholar, Science Direct, Scopus, and PubMed, were explored for key words including prevention programs, history, pandemic, and COVID-19 (Iranzadasl et al., 2021). Previous to April 2020, data published was collected along with traditional and modern information that was compared and analyzed. Data was coded and categorized into incoherent, preventive, and historical groupings (Iranzadasl et al., 2021).

Recurring items and codes were collected into common themes presented in tables and text. Significant contradictions were not evident in the study from the recommendations of traditional Persian physicians and recent protocols for pandemic control. The researchers recommended that variables such as strengthening the temperament, body cleansing, and nutrition may be overlooked in the current research for dealing with COVID-19. Finally, the researchers recommended evaluating the cumulative and multifactor effects of these variables (Iranzadasl et al., 2021).

Phenomenology Dissertation

In a dissertation study conducted by Burleson (2017), the main purpose was to determine multiple aspects supporting fundamental conditions of an efficacious integrative healthcare model in the United States. A phenomenology design captures the lived experiences of integrative healthcare practitioners to explore a better comprehension of essential factors and interactions guiding an effective integrative healthcare model. The researcher sought to provide relevant information for the leadership, management, and creation of effective integrative healthcare applications (Burleson, 2017). Furthermore, the researcher sought to understand the following areas:

- Healthcare relationship with patients,
- Approaches and treatments based upon science,
- Patient care coordination throughout all areas of patient care and wellbeing, and
- A prosperous integrative healthcare business model (Burleson, 2017).

A systems science perspective, in addition to a phenomenology design, directed the study. Encounters with patient and integrative healthcare practioners were explored. Moreover, impacts on staff, patients, and patient families were examined. Research questions addressed how practitioners characterize experiences when providing integrative services and how those experiences embody necessary variables related to successful best practices in the field of integrative healthcare (Burleson, 2017).

Four themes materialized from the research that included the following characteristics:

- The affect to wellbeing and health of the integrative healthcare practitioner,
- Best practices related to approached and requirements,
- The patient – practitioner relationship,
- The value of the practioners' professional journey in the field of integrative healthcare (Burleson, 2017).

Conclusion

This discussion analyzed four journal articles published in Integrative Medicine Research, volume 10, issue 1, March 2021. The discussion analyzed three systematic reviews and one qualitative design. In addition, one dissertation study was summarized regarding multiple aspects supporting fundamental conditions of an efficacious integrative healthcare model in the United States.

Integrative Healthcare Research

Corp, Jordan, and Croft (2018) examined 1486 justifications for the use of complementary and alternative medicine (CAM) from 169 papers documenting 152 different studies. Eleven specific categories over four themes included individuals' philosophy of care and illness, non-clinical outcomes of care, practical aspects of care, and clinical effectiveness (Corp et al., 2018). Individuals described common rationales for avoiding and using CAM. In addition, statements emphasized that CAM aligned with ideas and a general philosophy held by individuals regarding healthcare and illness. Moreover, collected statements expressed that CAM has the ability to give individuals control over one's treatment and condition (Corp et al., 2018).

Findings concluded that CAM appears to have a considerable role in offering choices to enable meeting the needs of individuals with painful, long-term, and common conditions (Corp et al., 2018). Of the 1486 justifications for the use of CAM extracted from the papers, discontinuation, continuation, and barriers to CAM use highlighted influences from conventional medicine (Corp et al., 2018). Influences included both positive, for example, a specific CAM therapy proposed by a doctor, and negative, for example, perceived ineffectiveness of conventional medicine treatment compelling the use of CAM (Corp et al., 2018).

The eleven categorical themes established regarding reasons individuals seek CAM interventions included the following:

- therapeutic environment,
- healthcare satisfaction,
- referral,
- how a condition is presented,
- safety,
- goal,
- effect,
- desperation,
- more healthcare control,
- confidence,
- accessibility, and
- convenience (Corp, et al., 2018).

Sociological, historical, and cultural phenomenon results of CAM studies emphasize the benefit of choice for healthcare users (Corp, et al., 2018). Patients reported using CAM with a high volume of satisfaction and use making these convictions an evident challenge to a conventional medicine system that only authorizes CAM usage if biomedical science and concepts are applied (Corp, et al., 2018). Barriers to CAM use included a lack of public awareness, understanding, education, knowledge, and incorrect stereotypes regarding CAM therapies, practitioners, and effectiveness (Corp, et al., 2018).

Further challenges included allopathic and pharmaceutical business structural barriers, lack of allopathic practitioner support, lack of formal referrals from allopathic practitioners, and lack of information regarding where to obtain treatment for CAM use (Corp, et al., 2018). Extensive studies with 1486 justifications including facilitators and barriers for CAM collected by these researchers identifies an elevated need for public education about CAM service providers, practitioners, treatments, therapies, use, and opportunities.

In a study conducted by the University of Arizona Integrative Health Center (UAIHC), outcomes reported by patients on various standardized measures and pre-post evaluation results concluded significant statistical improvements under continuous integrative primary care (Crocker, Hurwitz, Grizzle, Abraham, Rehfeld, Horwitz, Weil, & Maizes, 2019). After one year of integrative medicine (IM) primary care, positive patient improvement areas included physical activity, overall well-being, fatigue, pain, sleep quality, work productivity, physical, mental, and overall health (Crocker, et al., 2019).

One hundred seventy seven patients submitted baseline and follow-up outcome measurements and reported improvements in all areas except work absenteeism and perceived stress. IM was delivered in a primary healthcare model by UAIHC that blended complementary and conventional medical treatments that included groups, educational classes, health coaching, manual medicine, acupuncture, mind-body medicine, and nutrition (Crocker, et al., 2019). The overall health-related outcome measured for quality of life.

Reasons commonly cited in the study by patients for seeking IM care from UAIHC included the desire to avert an afflictive health condition and to expand wellbeing regardless of whether patients' illness was curable (Crocker, et al., 2019). Eighty-six percent of patients participating in the study were highly educated with a four-year college degree or higher, 70% female, 86% Caucasian, and 75% employed (Crocker, et al., 2019). UAIHC patients reported positive changes succeeding twelve months of IM care indicated that positive potential effects on patient outcomes when using IM approaches included well-being, work productivity, and quality of life. The study suggested that an educated public, when knowledgeable about IM approaches, could make informed decisions regarding healthcare options to improve overall health and wellbeing in various categories significant to quality of life.

Khorsan (2017) presented findings regarding identified perceived barriers and facilitators of integrative health care (IHC). The study was designed as a program evaluation over two years and was performed at an academic, university-based, medical clinic and center for IHC. In addition, the study examined potential successful models of IHC integration. Khorsan designed a mixed methodology using qualitative interviews and observations with significant stakeholders, healthcare providers, and patients. Quantitative results included responses by participants to a patient satisfaction scale and demographic data.

Identified themes included external barriers for IHC such as insurance regulations and payment. Other structural barriers included costs. Facilitators for actualization IHC included knowledge and empathy exchange, communication to foster trust, culture, and shared values. Furthermore, team-based and collaborative approaches can influence an IHC design and evolutionary path. Khorsan (2017) found that although some indicators of IHC integration were evident, considerable difficulties continue to persist preventing IHC providers from functioning as hospital providers in an academic-based context.

Notable themes in the study determined that a change strategy with interdisciplinary integration is important to engage IHC providers in mainstream trans-disciplinary research, education, and healthcare opportunities (Khorsan, 2017). Wider political and structural barriers continue to persist and obstruct successful IHC integration. The study bears important themes consistent to the notion that structural barriers and bias factors continue to marginalize and exclude IHC models and IHC practitioners from research, education, and healthcare opportunities. These barriers ultimately affect public health and public healthcare education when bias, exclusion, and significant structural barriers endure.

Public health is negatively affected by limited, scarce, and unavailable integrative healing opportunities and education. Public health is further marginalized by many traditional health insurance models that refuse to cover the costs of integrative healing alternatives and providers. The literature review synthesized research supporting alternative medicine and healthcare opportunities for overall improved health and wellbeing.

Four themes materialized from the research that included the following characteristics:

- The affect to wellbeing and health of the integrative healthcare practitioner,
- Best practices related to approached and requirements,
- The patient – practitioner relationship,
- The value of the practioners' professional journey in the field of integrative healthcare (Burleson, 2017).

The literature review synthesized research supporting alternative medicine and healthcare options and opportunities for overall improved health and wellbeing. Furthermore, the research presented suggested that when the public is educated and knowledgeable about the benefits of alternative holistic medicine, the public can make more informed healthcare decisions in addition to seeking out how and where to find appropriate services, providers, therapies, and treatments.

About the Author

Dr. Lisa Marie Portugal holds a PhD in Leadership for Higher Education, an EdD in Public Health Education, a Master of Education in Educational Business Administration – Human Resources, a Master of Education in Health and Wellness, a Master of Arts in Education, and a Bachelor of Fine Arts. She completed 42 credits in a Doctor of Management (DM) in Executive Leadership program. She is a personal and professional life coach, author, university professor, PhD chair, committee member, and a faculty supervisor / mentor to teacher candidates. She currently instructs coursework at the undergraduate, graduate, EdD, and PhD levels for various universities and abroad. She is a researcher, peer–reviewed scholar, and educator. Dr. Portugal is on the review board for various academic journals. Her expertise and research interests include: Virtuous Leadership, Cultural Magnanimity, health and wellness, student engagement and success, student retention, adult learning theory, adult, nontraditional, and at–risk learners, faculty retention, hiring practices, faculty burn–out, best practices in online learning, emerging technology in course design and instruction, online education, learning styles, diversity leadership, and the Community of Inquiry Framework. She integrates theory into practice through conducting research in these areas.

Contact

Email:
lisamarieportugal@msn.com

Website:
http://drlisamarieportugal.weebly.com

Website:
https://drlisamarieportugal.wixsite.com/leadershiparchitect

Appendix

Bandura's Social Cognitive Theory

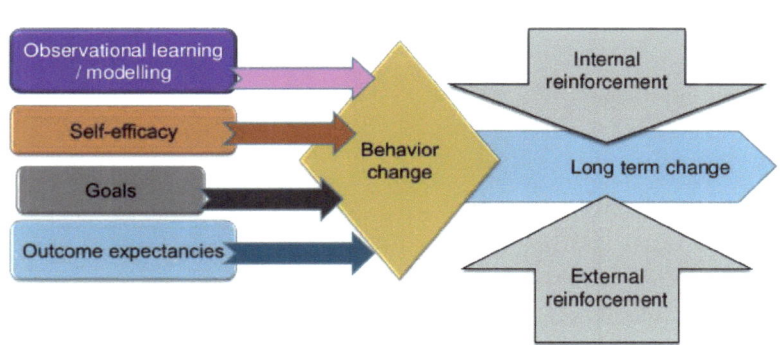

Adapted from Bandura, A. (1998). Health promotion from the perspective of social cognitive theory. *Psychology and Health, 13*. 623-649.

Determining Human Behavior with Social Cognitive Theory

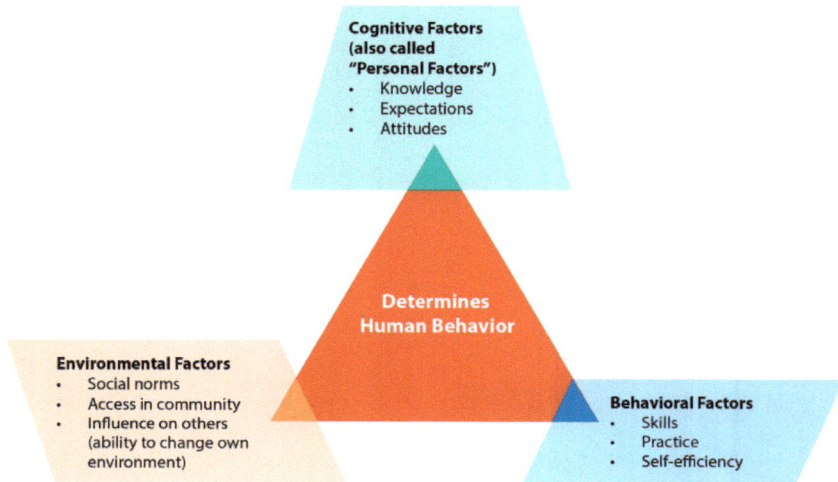

Adapted from Johns Hopkins University. (2016). *Annex A: Key SBCC theories in FP*.
https://sbccimplementationkits.org/htsp/annex-a-key-sbcc-theories-in-fp/

Social Cognitive Theory and Cognitive Behavior Modification

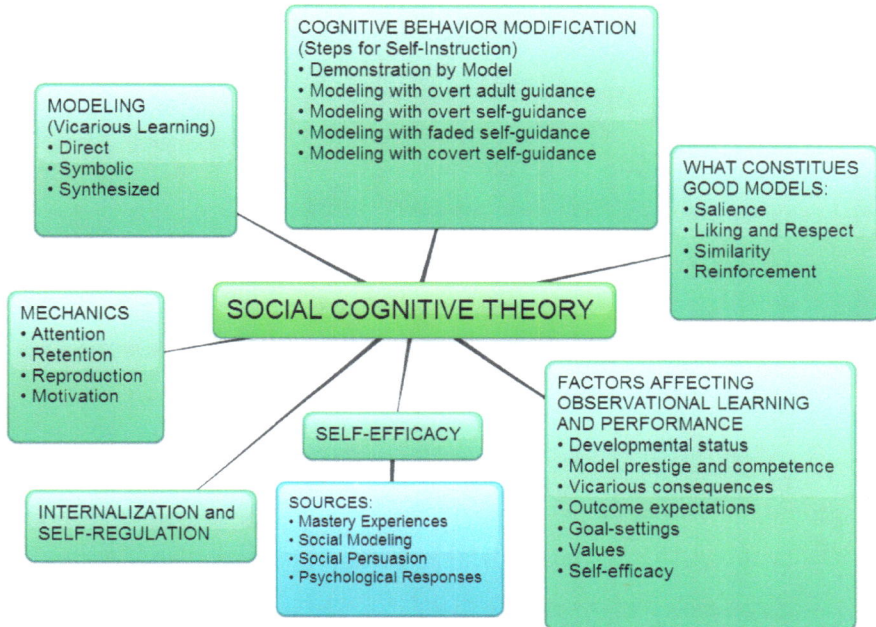

Adapted from Learning to Teach. Teaching to Learn. UPOU E-Journal. (2014, March 19). *Notes and resources*. https://owelpapel.wordpress.com/tag/notes-and-resources/

Self-Efficacy and Social Cognitive Theory

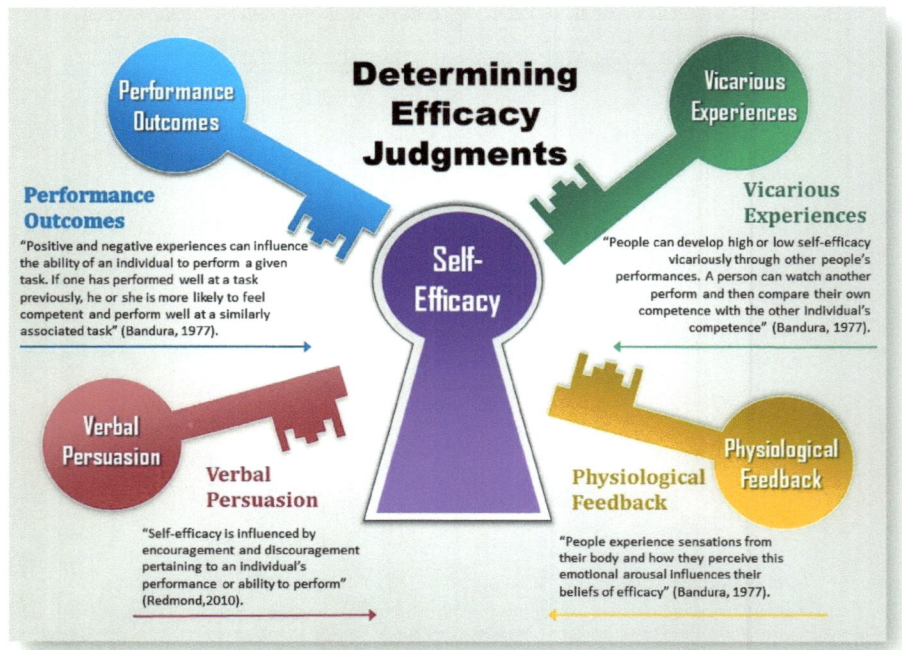

Adapted from Tinsley, A. L. (2017, April 12). *Spring 2016 ~ Self-efficacy and Social Cognitive Theories: Social Cognitive Theory and self-efficacy.* https://wikispaces.psu.edu/display/484SU17001/Spring+2016+~+Self-Efficacy+and+Social+Cognitive+Theories

References

Acharya, A., Blackwell, M. & Sen, S. (2018). Explaining attitudes from behavior: A cognitive dissonance approach. *Journal of Politics 80*(2), 400-411. https://j.mp/2nzw6SY

Agunbiade, S. R. (2019). *Increase in Americans use of complementary and alternative medicines: A qualitative case study of use of herbal medicine in New York City* (Publication No. 13902110) [Doctoral dissertation, University of Phoenix]. ProQuest Dissertations and Thesis and Global.

Ali, A. & Katz, D. L. (2015, November). Disease prevention and health promotion: How integrative medicine fits. *American Journal of Preventive Medicine, 49*(5), S230-S240. Retrieved from https://doi.org/10.1016/j.amepre.2015.07.019

Ang, L., Lee, H. W., Choi, J. Y., Zhang, J., & Lee, M. S. (2020, June). Herbal medicine and pattern identification for treating COVID-19: A rapid review of guidelines. *Integrative Medicine Research, 9*(2).

Ang, L., Lee, H. W., Kim, A., Lee, J. A., & Lee, M. S. (2020, May). Herbal medicine for treatment of children diagnosed with COVID-19: A review of guidelines. *Complementary Therapies in Clinical Practice, 39*.

Bandura, A. (1998). Health promotion from the perspective of social cognitive theory. *Psychology and Health, 13*. 623-649.

Bandura, A. (2004, April). Health promotion by social cognitive means. *Health Education & Behavior, 31*(2). 143-164. Retrieved from http://www.uky.edu/~eushe2/Bandura/Bandura2004HEB.pdf

Belil, F. E., Alhani, F., Ebadi, A., & Kazemnejad, A. (2018, November 3). Self-efficacy of people with chronic conditions: A qualitative directed content analysis. *Journal of Clinical Medicine, 7*(11), 411.

Bensley, R. J., & Brookins-Fisher, J (2019). *Community and public health education methods* (4th ed.). Jones & Bartlett Learning.

Burleson, D. (2017). *The dynamic interactions of an integrative healthcare experience: A phenomenological study through the lived experiences of integrative healthcare professionals* (Doctoral dissertation). Retrieved from Retrieved from ProQuest Dissertations and Theses Global database. (10624624)

Chan, A., Tay, H. L., Shih, V., Tan, H. C., & Chiang, J. (2012). Clinical outcomes for cancer patients using complementary and alternative medicine. *Alternative Therapies in Health and Medicine, 18*(1), 12-17.

Chin, J. H., & Mansori, S. (2019) Theory of Planned Behaviour and Health Belief Model: Females' intention on breast cancer screening. *Cogent Psychology, 6*(1).

Chu, X., Sun, B., Huang, Q., & Zhang, Y. (2020, May). Preference degree-based multi-granularity sequential three-way group conflict decisions approach to the integration of TCM and Western medicine. *Computers & Industrial Engineering, 143.*

Chunga, V. C. H., Wong, C. H. L., Zhong, C. C. W., Tjioe, Y. Y., Leung, T. H., & Griffiths, S. M. (2021, March). Traditional and complementary medicine for promoting healthy ageing in WHO Western Pacific Region: Policy implications from utilization patterns and current evidence. *Integrative Medicine Research, 10*(1). https://doi.org/10.1016/j.imr.2020.100469

Conley, C. E. W., Olson, A. D., Howard, J. S., Dressler, E. V., Lattermann, C., & Mattacola, C. G (2018). Use of an adaption to the health belief model to influence rehabilitation adherence in athletic training. *Athletic Training and Sports Health Care. 10*(1), 10-19.

Corp, N., Jordan, J. L., & Croft, P. R. (2018, July 19). Justifications for using complementary and alternative medicine reported by persons with musculoskeletal conditions: A narrative literature synthesis. *Plos One, 13*(7), e0200879. Retrieved from https://doi.org/10.1371/journal.pone.0200879

Cottrell, R. R., Girvan, J. T., McKenzie, J. F., & Seabert, D. (2018). *Principles and foundations of health promotion and education* (7th ed.). Pearson.

Crocker, R. L., Hurwitz, J. T., Grizzle, A. J., Abraham, I., Rehfeld, R., Horwitz, R., Weil, A. T., & Maizes, V. (2019). Real-world evidence from the integrative medicine primary care trial (impact): Assessing patient-reported outcomes at baseline and 12-month follow-up. *Evidence-Based Complementary & Alternative Medicine (ECAM)*, 1-9. https://doi.org/10.1155/2019/8595409

Doyle, E. I., Ward, S. E., & Early, J. (2019). *The process of community health education and promotion* (3rd ed.). Waveland Press.

Gerontakos, S., Casteleijn, D., & Wardlea, J. (2021, March). Clinician perspectives and understanding of the adaptogenic concept: A focus group study with Naturopaths and Western Herbalists. *Integrative Medicine Research, 10*(1). https://doi.org/10.1016/j.imr.2020.100433

Glanz, K., Rimer, B. K., & Lewis, F. M. (2002). *Health behavior and health education: Theory, research and practice.* Wiley & Sons.

Harmon-Jones, E. (2012). Cognitive Dissonance Theory. In: V. S. Ramachandran (ed). *The Encyclopedia of Human Behavior, 1.* 543-549. Academic Press. Elsevier, Inc.

Ho, L. T. F., Chan, K. K. H., Chung, V. C. H., & Leung, T. H. (2020, June). Highlights of traditional Chinese medicine frontline expert advice in the China national guideline for COVID-19. *European Journal of Integrative Medicine, 36.*

Hung, M., Ekwueme, D. U., White, A., Rim, S. H., & Chang, S. (2018, January). Estimating health benefits and cost-savings for achieving the Healthy People 2020 objective of reducing invasive colorectal cancer. *Preventive Medicine, 106*, 38-44.

Integrative Health Practitioner. (2019). *The 7 integrative disciplines of IHP*. Retrieved from https://www.integrativehealthpractitioner.org/?msclkid=fb691f78883c1f665c8a407bf2c607da&utm_source=bing&utm_medium=cpc&utm_campaign=Apply%20Now&utm_term=%2Bintegrative%20%2Bhealthcare&utm_content=Integrative%20health%20practitioner%20BMM

Iranzadasl, M., Karimi, Y., Moadeli, F., & Pasalar, M. (2021, March). Persian medicine recommendations for the prevention of pandemics related to the respiratory system: a narrative literature review. *Integrative Medicine Research, 10*(1). https://doi.org/10.1016/j.imr.2020.100483

Kennedy, D. A., Lupattelli, A., Koren, G., & Nordeng, H. (2016). Safety classification of herbal medicines used in pregnancy in a multinational study. *BMC Complementary and Alternative Medicine, 16*.

Kim, C., Sung, K., Kim, D., Chu, H., & Lee, S. (2020, March). Development of integrative medicine therapy for gastrointestinal autoimmune diseases: A study protocol for a registry study. *Integrative Medicine Research, 9*(1), 65-71.

Khorsan, R. (2017). *A program evaluation of an academic integrative healthcare center: Barriers to, and facilitators in, applying integrative medicine to primary care* (Publication No. 10688980) [Doctoral dissertation, University of Phoenix]. ProQuest Dissertations and Thesis and Global.

Kircher, C., Watson-Whitmyre, M., & Montvilo, R. K. (2008). *Herbal medicine* (4th ed.). Hackensack, NJ: Salem.

LaMorte, W. W. (2016, April 28). Behavioral change models: The social cognitive theory. *Boston University School of Public Health.* Retrieved from http://sphweb.bumc.bu.edu/otlt/MPH-Modules/SB/BehavioralChangeTheories/BehavioralChangeTheories5.html

Ling, C., Fan, J., Lin, H., & Shen, F. (2018, July). Clinical practice guidelines for the treatment of primary liver cancer with integrative traditional Chinese and Western medicine. *Journal of Integrative Medicine, 16*(4), 236-248.

McAlister, A. L., Perry, C. L., & Parcel, G. S. (2008). How individuals, environments, and health behaviors interact: Social cognitive theory. *In Glanz, K., Rimer, B. K., Viswanath, K. Health behavior and health education: Theory, research, and practice* (4th ed.). Jossey-Bass.

Mehl-Madova, L, Managny, B., & Plummer, J. (2016). Integration of complementary and alternative medicine therapies into primary care pain management for opiate reduction in a rural setting. *The journal of Alternative and Complementary Medicine, 22*(8) 621 -626.

National Institutes of Health (NIH). (2020, May 27). Opioid overdose crisis. *U.S. Department of Health and Human Services.* https://www.drugabuse.gov/drug-topics/opioids/opioid-overdose-crisis

Ng, J. Y., Nault, H., & Nazir, Z. (2021, March). Complementary and integrative medicine mention and recommendations: A systematic review and quality assessment of lung cancer clinical practice guidelines. *Integrative Medicine Research, 10*(1). https://doi.org/10.1016/j.imr.2020.100452

RDM NEWSWIRE. (2015, November 5). *Health council in 'state of multi-system' failure.* https://www.sowetanlive.co.za/news/2015-11-05-health-council-in-state-of-multi-system-failure/

RegisteredNursing.org. (2020, June 28). *What is integrative healthcare?* Retrieved from https://www.registerednursing.org/what-integrative-healthcare/

Schunk, D. H., & DiBenedetto, M. K. (2020, January). Motivation and social cognitive theory. *Contemporary Educational Psychology, 60.* https://doi.org/10.1016/j.cedpsych.2019.101832

Sell, K., Amella, E., Mueller, M., Andrews, J., & Wachs, J. (2016) Use of Social Cognitive Theory to assess salient clinical research in chronic disease self-management for older adults: An integrative review. *Open Journal of Nursing, 6.* 213-228. https://www.scirp.org/journal/PaperInformation.aspx?PaperID=64944

Tan, C-E. (2014, October 11). *Health behaviour and health education for family medicine postgraduates.* https://www.slideshare.net/ChaiEngTan/health-behaviour-and-health-education-for-family-medicine-postgraduates-40155488

Tougas, M. E., Hayden, J. A., McGrath, P. J., Huguet, A., & Rozario, S. (2015, August 7). A systematic review exploring the social cognitive theory of self-regulation as a framework for chronic health condition interventions. *PLoS ONE, 10*(8), e0134977. Retrieved from https://doi.org/10.1371/journal.pone.0134977

Tomlinson, C. A. (2017). *How to differentiate instruction in academically diverse classrooms. (3rd ed.).* ASCD.

van Geel, M., Keuning, T., Frèrejean, J., Dolmans, D., van Merriënboer, J., & Visscher, A. J. (2019) Capturing the complexity of differentiated instruction. *School Effectiveness and School Improvement, 30*(1), 51-67. https://www.tandfonline.com/doi/full/10.1080/09243453.2018.1539013

Westchester Wellness Medicine Transforme MD. (2020). *Integrative medicine.* https://www.westchesterwellnessmedicine.com/integrative-medicine.html

Whitley, J., Gooderham, S., Duquette, C., Orders, S., & Cousins, J. B. (2019) Implementing differentiated instruction: A mixed-methods exploration of teacher beliefs and practices. *Teachers and Teaching, 25*(8), 1043-1061. https://www.tandfonline.com/doi/abs/10.1080/13540602.2019.1699782

Witt, C. (2017, March 20). A new definition of integrative health. *The Institute for Integrative Health (TIIH)*. Retrieved from https://tiih.org/who/blog/new-definition-integrative-health/

World Health Organization (WHO). (2012). *The WHO regional strategy for traditional medicine in the Western Pacific Region (2011-2020)*. http://www.wpro.who.int/publications/2012/regionalstrategyfortraditionalmedicine_2012.pdf

World Health Organization. (WHO). (2013). *Intro 5. WHO traditional medicine strategy (2014-2023)*. http://apps.who.int/iris/bitstream/10665/92455/1/9789241506090_eng.pdf

Ziodeen, K. A. & Misra, S. M. (2018, April). Complementary and integrative medicine attitudes and perceived knowledge in a large pediatric residency program. *Complementary Therapies in Medicine, 37*, 133-135. https://doi.org/10.1016/j.ctim.2018.02.004

Cover image from Westchester Wellness Medicine Transforme MD. (2020). *Integrative medicine*. https://www.westchesterwellnessmedicine.com/integrative-medicine.html

First page image from RDM NEWSWIRE. (2015, November 5). *Health council in 'state of multi-system' failure*. https://www.sowetanlive.co.za/news/2015-11-05-health-council-in-state-of-multi-system-failure/

Page 6 image from Herbal Medicine. https://www.complementarytherapiesnewmills.co.uk/herbal-medicine/

www.ingramcontent.com/pod-product-compliance
Lightning Source LLC
Chambersburg PA
CBHW040224220526
45473CB00001B/110